Emanuella Pinheiro de Farias Bispo
Carlos H. F. Tavares
Jerzuí Mendes Tôrres Tomaz

Interdisciplinarity in Health Teaching:

Emanuella Pinheiro de Farias Bispo
Carlos H. F. Tavares
Jerzuí Mendes Tôrres Tomaz

Interdisciplinarity in Health Teaching:

The preceptor's view in the Family Health Strategy

ScienciaScripts

Imprint

Cover image: Provided by the author

This book is a translation from the original published under ISBN 978-3-330-20273-3.

Publisher:
Sciencia Scripts
is a trademark of
Dodo Books Indian Ocean Ltd. and OmniScriptum S.R.L publishing group

120 High Road, East Finchley, London, N2 9ED, United Kingdom
Str. Armeneasca 28/1, office 1, Chisinau MD-2012, Republic of Moldova, Europe
Printed at: see last page
ISBN: 978-620-8-30077-7

INDICE

Chapter 1	3
Chapter 2	6
Chapter 3	20
Chapter 4	45
Chapter 5	56

SUMMARY

This paper presents an article entitled "Interdisciplinarity in Health Teaching: The Family Health Perspective", which aimed to analyze how interdisciplinarity is used by preceptors in the health supports of the Family Health Strategies of the II Sanitary District of Maceio. To interpret and analyze the data, the "open or in-depth interview" data collection instrument was used, from the perspective of *Content Analysis.* The data from this study showed that the subjects were unaware of interdisciplinarity. Based on the results of this research, a product was developed in the form of an intervention project entitled: "Interdisciplinarity in Health Teaching: Reframing collective support through a shared and integrated approach". The aim of this product is to train the professional preceptors of the II Health District of Maceio in the theory and practice of interdisciplinary Family Health Strategies. Preceptors are the main multipliers of interdisciplinary support in their Family Health teams and are present in the training of students in the perspective of interdisciplinarity. We therefore believe that *Interdisciplinarity* can help overcome the dissociation of the knowledge produced and guide the production of a new order of knowledge, constituting a necessary condition for improving training in Health for the Unified Health System (SUS).

Keywords: Preceptor. Interdisciplinary Health Team. Family Health Program.

1 PRESENTATION

This work is the result of my personal and professional career, above all, my training and work in interdisciplinarity, in order to understand the obstacles and new possibilities for building knowledge in the field of health teaching.

One of the National Constitution's guidelines for health supports and services, when they are constituted as a single system, is comprehensive care, i.e. comprehensive care as a constitutional principle guiding the formulation of health policies. For this to happen, interdisciplinary support is needed to guide training and health policies. As far as training is concerned, the preceptor is a professional who is not from the academy but from the service, with higher education in the health area and who receives students in the practice settings of Higher Education Institutions.

The Family Health Strategy (ESF) is an important instrument for operationalizing health support geared towards what is recommended by the Unified Health System (SUS). The ESF preceptor has a very relevant differential, which is the fact that he or she is in a field that in itself enables a broader view of health, through shared, collective and integrated practices. These practices enable new perspectives and new paths within health education.

Considering the importance of the figure of the preceptor in narrowing the gap between theory and practice in the training of students, this study sought to analyze how interdisciplinarity is instrumentalized by preceptors in the health supports of the Family Health Strategies (ESF) of the II Sanitary District of Maceio.

This is a final paper in the Professional Master's Program in Health Teaching at the Faculty of Medicine (FAMED) of the Federal University of Alagoas (UFAL). It presents research in the form of an article entitled "Interdisciplinarity in Health Teaching: The Preceptor's View of the Family Health Strategy" and an intervention project entitled "Interdisciplinarity in Health Teaching: Re-signifying collective support through a shared and integrated view", the aim of which is to train the professional preceptors of the II Health District of Maceio in interdisciplinarity.

Both the scientific article and the intervention project are the result of in-depth theoretical and field research in the area of Health Teaching, with *interdisciplinarity* as the main object of study.

The article is a field study and we opted for the *open-ended or in-depth interview* technique, from the perspective of Content Analysis for data analysis. The theoretical framework used was interdisciplinarity, health teaching from the perspective of the Unified Health System (SUS) and the Family Health Strategy. The study was submitted to Interface - Comunicapao, Saude, Educapao, an interdisciplinary journal.

The article presents data from a survey that revealed how professional preceptors act in terms of *interdisciplinarity.* One of the results of this study was that the subjects were distanced from what characterizes interdisciplinary theory and practice. The product, based on the results obtained, is characterized by a proposal for an intervention, in the form of training, on the theory and practice of *interdisciplinarity.* The target audience for the training are the subjects of this research. The product will be offered to the Higher Education Institution involved in partnership with the Municipal Health Department, with the aim of training the professional preceptors of the II Sanitary District of Maceio in the theory and practice of interdisciplinary Family Health Strategy.

The findings of this study are presented and broken down below.

2. INTERDISCIPLINARITY IN HEALTH TEACHING: A REFLECTION ON CONCEPTS, OBSTACLES AND NEW PERSPECTIVES

SUMMARY

This research, based on a literature review, invites reflection on the importance of discussing interdisciplinarity in the area of health teaching. It is a theoretical study based on a critical review of the literature on the highlighted context. The texts were searched for in the databases of the Virtual Health Library (Lilacs - Index of Scientific and Technical Literature of Latin America and the Caribbean and Scielo - Scientific Electronic Library Online). By reading the manuscripts obtained, it was possible to construct a reflective synthesis on the subject. It is therefore considered that interdisciplinarity can help to overcome the dissociation of the knowledge produced and guide the production of a new order of scientific knowledge, which is a necessary condition for improving health training for the Unified Health System (SUS), by trying to overcome fragmentation. Since their training, health professionals must move towards integrating knowledge within the process of forming care networks. Occupational Therapy is no different. This professional, whose essence is to see the individual from various aspects within their complexity, needs training that accompanies this profile for interdisciplinary practice.

DESCRIPTORS: Interdisciplinarity, Health Teaching, Education.

2.1 Introduction

Critics of education agree that the biologicist, medicalizing and procedure-centered approach of health professionals is hegemonic. They suffer from the advance of specializations, which results in the dismantling of knowledge and the fragmentation of man. Likewise, health is an increasingly complex field and the depth of scientific knowledge and technical advances are not enough to deal with this complexity. Interdisciplinarity therefore presents itself as a possible solution to these issues, facilitating a broader approach to man, with the aim of overcoming the critical problems of the past, giving way to the benefits of a new health practice (Guedes, 2010). In most cases, this health practice is found within a hegemonic pedagogical model of teaching, which encourages early specialization and perpetuates traditional models of health practice (Feuerwerker, 2002 apud Ceccim, 2004).

In this way, the National Curriculum Guidelines (DCN's) for undergraduate health courses of 2001 and 2002 state that the training of health professionals should take into account "the *health system in force in the country, teamwork* and *comprehensive health care",* reaffirming the practice of orientation towards the Unified Health System (SUS) (Almeida, 2003 apud Ceccim 2004). Ceccim (2004), in turn, talks about curricular changes and argues that the university is responsible for training professionals who establish a *reciprocal* relationship with society. In this way, the Ministry of Health and Education are making efforts to transform the organization of health services and training processes with a focus on reorienting the current care model.

In this context, as Japiassu (1976) states, *"the conduct of one disciplinary organization passes through the conduct of the other, and vice versa, and both conducts change, modify each other reciprocally", we* think of the need for an interdisciplinary, unified and convergent vision, implied in being present in both the field of theory and practice, whether this practice is social intervention, pedagogy or research (Gattas, 2006).

The aim of this study is to describe, explain and analyze the phenomena related to interdisciplinary teaching in health, since there is a need to broaden the dialogue on the importance of theoretical and practical knowledge of this subject.

2.2 Methods

This is a theoretical study based on a critical review of the literature. The texts were searched in the databases of the Virtual Health Library: Lilacs (Index of Scientific and Technical Literature of Latin America and the Caribbean) and Scielo (Scientific Electronic Library Online). The inclusion criteria for this search were: publication between 2000 and 2014; texts in Portuguese; search descriptors: "Interdisciplinarity", "Teaching in Health" and "Education". By crossing these three descriptors, the texts were organized to construct a reflective summary of the topic.

2.3 Results and Discussion

Some authors point to various meanings of what could be called the phenomenon of interdisciplinarity. This phenomenon can be seen as an epistemological theory or as a methodological proposal for pedagogical action or scientific research (Paviane, 2003). It can also be characterized as a conceptual, theoretical and methodological exchange, as well as an application of knowledge from one discipline to another (Paviane, 2003; Japiassu, 1976).

Japiassu argues that we go through successive degrees of increasing cooperation and coordination before reaching the interdisciplinary level. This can be characterized as a level at which collaboration between different disciplines or between heterogeneous sectors of the same science leads to actual interaction, i.e. reciprocal exchanges, so that at the end of the interactive process, each discipline is enriched.

The extreme fragmentation of knowledge has placed interdisciplinarity at the center of discussions about the development of science and health practices (Matos et al, 2009). It is true that there are obstacles to be overcome. Japiassu (1976) says that these obstacles are "stumbling blocks" that prevent the concrete realization of valid and effective collaboration between disciplines. It is true that there are obstacles to be overcome. One of these "stumbling blocks" may be the influence of the fragmented model of work organization, in which each professional carries out parts of their work without integrating it with the other areas involved (Matos, 2009; Japiassu, 1976). This is one of the reasons why it is difficult to achieve a more integrated and better quality health service, both from the perspective of those who carry it out and those who benefit from it (Matos, 2009). Interdisciplinarity can thus be seen as an attempt to tackle the excessive fragmentation of knowledge and not just as a way of integrating and collaborating teachers or researchers (Paviane, 2003). So wouldn't we first have to know the meaning of the disciplines in order to then understand what motivates them to come together?

According to Japiassu (1976), talking about interdisciplinary methodology means, first and foremost, talking about operating and cooperating disciplines. Initially, a discipline must develop its own concepts and ensure that these are as operative as possible, acquiring their own unity, their own law. After this stage, it can cooperate with other disciplines.

You know that trying to "break down barriers" can be done at different levels. The first is the level of juxtaposition, of parallelism, where the various disciplines are there but do not interact. On the second level, the disciplines communicate with each other, reconfront and discuss their perspectives. On the third level, they overcome the barriers that have kept them apart, merging into something new that transcends them all. Interdisciplinarity would therefore designate the space *in between* these moments.

mentioned (Pombo, 2004).

Even though it is an obstacle to be overcome, interdisciplinarity is increasingly becoming a necessity, a condition of epistemological possibility and the fundamental politics of knowledge (Paviane, 2003). Interdisciplinary practice can increase the chances of health training that is more critical and more in tune with the needs of the population, presupposing new forms of relationship with regard to the relationships that workers establish between themselves and with service users, with the aim of establishing bridges between initially antagonistic positions (Gattas, 2006; Paviane, 2003; Furtado, 2009).

It can be seen that interdisciplinarity is understood by many as a necessity imposed by the nature of research. On this issue, Furtado (2009) argues that the *logic of* professional *collaboration* is a need to share knowledge.

knowledge, specialties, experiences, skills and even intersubjectivity, which enables a broader understanding of the object of health work and an interaction of knowledge and actions (Furtado, 2009).

Within this discussion, we come to another term that intertwines interdisciplinarity: *integrality.* This is one of the basic guidelines of the Unified Health System (SUS), established by the 1988 Constitution. This became known as the Citizen's Constitution and was marked by the recognition of many citizenship rights, including health, which was recognized as a right for all and a duty of the state. In this context, Saupe et al (2005) state in their research that "interdisciplinarity is one of the elements, or one of the paths, that makes it possible to get closer to a Comprehensive Health Care practice".

Despite the progress made with the Unified Health System (SUS), its guiding principles are not yet a reality in health services (Linard, 2011). The search for a holistic approach cannot forgo an interdisciplinary vision/posture. This, in turn, implies an awareness of the limits and potential of each field of knowledge towards a collective approach (Garcia, 2006). It is a fact that professionals who seek to orient their practices around the principle of integrality systematically seek to escape reductionism (Mattos, 2001). Thus, a new model of comprehensive health care, based on the principles and guidelines of the Unified Health System (SUS), requires professionals with technical and ethical competence, capable of understanding that *"the incidence of a single beam of light is not enough to illuminate an object"* (Japiassu, 1976), but that multiple focuses contribute to its understanding and appreciation (Garcia, 2006). The Family Health Strategy (ESF), created in 1994 as a proposal to review primary care practices, provides greater interaction between professionals and between professionals and users, creating a common territory that enables dialogue between subjects, generating a reorganization of care (Linard, 2011; Ferreira, 2011).

"To think about the collective dimension of health support is to affirm that health is not produced by a single being, but is born from the relationship with the other, from the way relationships happen." (Ferreira et al,2011, page 184). Interdisciplinarity seeks, through teamwork, the construction of new knowledge and the reconnection of knowledge with the aim of solving the user's need for comprehensive health care. Thus, compliance with the principle of comprehensiveness has become one of the greatest challenges facing healthcare in Brazil (Linard, 2011).

According to Fazenda (1994), *"perceiving oneself as interdisciplinary is the first movement towards interdisciplinary doing and interdisciplinary thinking"*. In order to do this, it is necessary to recognize the importance of interdisciplinary thinking, both during academic training and throughout professional life, as a way of practicing the connection between different types of knowledge. For this reason, the curricula of health courses can no longer be seen as a "neutral" set of knowledge and a mere division between the technical and human aspects involved in health training. It is necessary to overcome the dichotomized view of health teaching and build an integrative view of the training of health professionals, focusing mainly on interdisciplinarity (Ronzani, 2007).

Favarao and Araujo (2004) argue that today's society demands that universities not only train academics for future qualifications in traditional specializations, but above all, that they aim to train academics in health, to develop their skills and abilities in the light of new knowledge that is being produced and that requires a new type of professional.

Guedes and Ferreira Junior (2010) state that one of the main obstacles to interdisciplinarity identified in their study is the traditional training of different health professionals, which still values the fragmentation of knowledge and excessive specialization. In this regard, Bispo et al (2014) observed that the deficiency in academic and postgraduate training reflects the lack of preparation of academics for interdisciplinary practice of an integrative nature.

"In this way, education should be understood and worked on in an interdisciplinary way, in which the student is an active, committed, responsible agent, capable of planning their actions, taking responsibility, taking action in the face of facts and interacting in the environment in which they live, thus contributing to improving the teaching-learning process (Favarao & Araujo, 2004). Japiassu (1976) states that *"there is a demand linked to student demands against fragmented, artificially cut-off knowledge, because reality is global and multidimensional".* Thus, it can be seen that students need an education based on the integration of knowledge.

More et al. (2004) state that the interaction between the members of a health team raises various questions about the attitude of these professionals, especially with regard to common support, which can lead to fragmented health support. These authors suggest that "this reality has generated a need for training, in order to develop and work with multidisciplinary dialogues towards interdisciplinary ones". On this issue, Japiassu (1976) points to the need to improve and retrain teachers, reorienting them from specialized training to study aimed at solving problems by reorienting knowledge. Cotta (2006) mentions the qualification/training of health professionals as one of the ways to achieve higher quality health care services.

There is also a need to raise awareness of the recognition of interdisciplinary work and its importance for the training of future professionals for the Unified Health System (SUS). The first obstacle must be overcome: that of language (Japiassu, 1976). From there, we can build paths to collaboration, the construction of new areas of assistance, teaching, research and articulation with the community (Batista, 2005).

It is necessary for university curricula in the health area to promote interdisciplinarity by prioritizing elementary content and eliminating repetitive content (Favarao & Araujo, 2004). It is true that interdisciplinary work should be encouraged and prioritized whenever possible. Moving towards an integrated curriculum is a fundamental strategy for stimulating changes in training and, consequently, changes in health practice (Gonzalez, 2010). It is clear that interdisciplinary support can be practiced in higher education as long as there is a guideline in the pedagogical project, a teaching team committed to methodological innovation and institutional managers committed to making changes (Souza et al., 2012).

In their article, Almeida et al. (2012) report on the interdisciplinary support and strategies developed in health units by six undergraduate courses at the University of Fortaleza. These courses are: Physiotherapy, Pharmacy, Speech Therapy, Occupational Therapy, Physical Education and Nutrition. Despite the progress made, the courses need to establish the role of each profession in Primary Health Care, where the biggest challenge is to strengthen interdisciplinary action, including greater partnership with the Family Health Support Centers (NASF).

In this way, health courses must distance themselves from the logic of the medical-care-privatist model and seek to bring to their field of theoretical reflection and to their practical support a commitment to the objective and subjective needs of the population they serve, based on an expanded vision of health. To this end, it is essential to build an education based on the integration of knowledge and interprofessional practices in order to achieve this broader vision and integrated care.

2.4 Final considerations

Interdisciplinarity presents a possibility of overcoming the dissociation of scientific knowledge and seeks a new order of knowledge, constituting a necessary condition for improving health training for the Unified Health System (SUS).

It is well known that one of the university's functions is to produce new knowledge and apply it to social reality. It is therefore necessary to create restructuring strategies in health education in order to enable interdisciplinary communication within academic spaces and in a variety of training scenarios. To this end, the training and commitment of managers and teachers to this new interdisciplinary methodology is essential, justified by their responsibility for forming a graduate profile that meets the guidelines of the country's current health system.

REFERENCES

ALMEIDA, M. M. et al. From theory to practice of interdisciplinarity: the experience of Pro-Saude Unifor and its nine undergraduate courses. *Rev. bras. educ. rned.*[online]. 2012, vol.36, n.1, suppl.1, pp. 119-126.

ALMEIDA M, (org.). Diretrizes curriculares nacionais para os cursos universitárias da área da saúde. Londrina: Rede
Unida; 2003. In: Ceccim, R.B.; Feuerweker, L.C.M. Mudanpa na graduapao das profissoes de saude sob o eixo da integralidade. Cad. Saude Publica. Rio de Janeiro, v.20, n. 5, 2004.

BATISTA, SHS. Interdisciplinarity in medical education. Brazilian Journal of Medical Education. Rio de Janeiro, v.30, n.01, Jan-Apr, 2006.

BISPO, E. P. F. et al. Interdisciplinarity in health teaching: the preceptor's view of Family Health. *Interface (Botucatu)* [online]. 2014, vol.18, n.49, pp. 337-350. Epub Mar 10, 2014.

BRAZIL. Official Gazette of the Union. Law 8080/90. Provides for the conditions for the promotion, protection and recovery of health, the organization and financing of the corresponding services.
and other measures. Brasilia DF, September 19, 1990.

CECCIM, R.B.; FEUERWEKER, L.C.M. Mudanpa na graduapao das profissoes de saude sob o eixo da integralidade. Cad. Saude Publica v.20, n.5, Rio de Janeiro, Sept./Oct. 2004.

COTTA, R.M.M et al. Work organization and profile of Family Health Program professionals: a challenge in the restructuring of basic health care. Epidemiologia e Servipos de Saude. v. 15, n.3, p. 7 - 18, 2006.

FAVARAO, N.R.L; ARAUJO, C.S.A. Importance of the Interdisciplinarity in Higher Education. EDUCERE. Umuarama, v.4, n.2, p.103-115, jul./dez., 2004.

FAZENDA, IC. Interdisciplinarity: history, theory and research. Campinas: Papirus, 1994.

FERREIRA, RC; CHIRELLI, MQ; PEREIRA, AG. Psychological Approach in Primary Health Care: from Fragmentation to Integrality. Revista Brasileira de Educagao Medica. v. 35, n.2, p.177185, 2011.

FEUERWERKER LCM. Beyond the discourse of change in medical education: processes and results. Sao Paulo: Editora Hucitec/Londrina: Rede Unida/ Rio de Janeiro: Brazilian Association of Medical Education; 2002. In: Ceccim, R.B.; Feuerweker, L.C.M. Mudanga na graduação das profissoes de saude sob o eixo da integralidade. Cad. Saude Publica. v.20, n.5, Rio de Janeiro, Sept./Oct, 2004.

FURTADO, JP. Institutional Arrangements and Clinic Management: Principles of Interdisciplinarity and Interprofessionality. Cad. Bras. Saude Mental, v. 1, n. 1, jan-abr, 2009.

GARCIA, M.L.A *et al.* Interdisciplinarity and Integrality in Health Teaching. Rev. Cienc. Med., Campinas, v. 15, n.6, p.473-485, Nov./Dec., 2006.

GARCIA, M.L.A, *et al.* Interdisciplinarity Necessary for Medical Education. Revista Brasileira de Educagao Medica. v. 31, n.2, p.147 - 155; 2007.

GATTAS, M.L.G. Interdisciplinaridade - Formação e Agao na área de Saude. Ribeirao Preto: Holos Editora: 2006.

GUEDES, L.E, Junior M.F. Disciplinary Relations in a Teaching and Research Center for Health Promotion and Disease Prevention Practices. Sao Paulo. Rev. Saude Sociedade. 2010; v.19, n.2, p.260272.

GONZALEZ, A.D; ALMEIDA, M.J. Activating Change in Higher Education in Health: Difficulties and Strategies. Revista Brasileira de Educapao Medica. v. 34, n.2, p. 238-246, 2010.

JAPIASSU, H. Interdisciplinaridade e Pathologia do Saber. Rio de Janeiro: Imago Editora LTDA; 1976.

LINARD, A.G, Castro M.M, Cruz A.K.L. Integralidade da assistência na compreensão dos profissionais da Estrategia Saude da Familia. Rev Gaucha Enferm. v. 32, n.3, p. 546-53, Porto Alegre, 2011.

MATOS, E; PIRES, D.E.P; CAMPOS, G.W.S. Working relationships in interdisciplinary teams: contributions to the constitution of new forms of health work organization. Rev Bras Enferm, v. 62, n.6, p. 863-9, nov-dez, Brasilia, 2009.

MATTOS, R. A. The meanings of comprehensiveness: some reflections on values that deserve to be defended. In: PINHEIRO, R.; MATTOS, R.A. (Org.) Os sentidos da integralidade na atenpao e no cuidado a saude. Rio de Janeiro: UERJ/IMS: ABRASCO, 2001.

MORE, CLOO, *et al.* The social representations of the psychologist among residents of the family health program and the importance of interdisciplinarity. Rev Psicologia Hospitalar. v.1, n.1, p.59-75, 2004.

PAVIANE, J. Disciplinarity and Interdisciplinarity. International Seminar Interdisciplinarity, Humanism, University, Faculty of Letters, University of Porto, November 12-14, 2003.

POMBO, O. Interdisciplinaridade e Integrapao dos Saberes. Text of a conference presented at the "Luso-Brazilian Congress on Epistemology and Interdisciplinarity in Postgraduate Studies"; Porto Alegre: June, 2004.

RONZANI, T.M. Curricular Reform in Health Courses: What is the Role of Crenpas? Revista Brasileira de Educapao Medica. v.31, n.1, p.: 38 - 43; 2007.

SAUPE, R, *et al.* Competence of health professionals for interdisciplinary work. Interface - Comunic., Saude, Educ., v.9, n.18, p.521-36, set/dez, 2005.

SOUZA, M. C. A. et al. Interdisciplinarity in higher education: from image-objective to reality! *Rev. bras. educ. med.* [online]. 2012, vol.36, n.1, suppl.2, pp. 158-163.

3. INTERDISCIPLINARITY IN HEALTH TEACHING: THE PRECEPTOR'S VIEW OF THE FAMILY HEALTH STRATEGY

3.1 Introduction

The traditional pedagogical model of health teaching encourages early specialization, with training geared towards a biologicist and medicalizing approach (FEUERWERKER, 2002). Interdisciplinarity, then, presents itself as a possibility for a new approach, given that in-depth scientific knowledge and technical advances are not enough to satisfy the breadth of possibilities that the health area needs (GUEDES, 2010).

Japiassu (1976, p.118) states that in order to understand the meaning of "interdisciplinary" we need to know what "discipline" means. For this author, to speak of interdisciplinarity is to speak of the interaction of disciplines. A discipline has the same meaning as "science", as "disciplinarity", which is characterized by its mastery of the objects of study it deals with, by its specificities and by the way it predicts and explains phenomena.

Thus, interdisciplinarity is the coming together of different disciplines, whether from a pedagogical or epistemological perspective, to build new knowledge. This knowledge, in turn, is produced by the intersection of different knowledge/disciplines. An interdisciplinary vision must be present in both theory and practice, whether this practice involves social intervention, pedagogy or research (GATTAS, 2006; PAVIANE, 2003).

Another term linked to interdisciplinarity is "integrality", which is one of the guidelines of the Unified Health System (SUS), established by the 1988 Constitution. The SUS is organized around three guidelines:

decentralization; comprehensive care; and community participation (MATTOS, 2005; GARCIA, 2006; LINARD, CASTRO, CRUZ, 2011).

From the perspective of Health Education/SUS, the new National Curriculum Guidelines for undergraduate health courses state that the training of professionals in this area must take into account the health system in force in the country, teamwork and comprehensive health care, reaffirming the practice of SUS orientation (BRASIL, 2001a; BRASIL, 2001b; BRASIL, 2002a; BRASIL, 2002b).

And the university, in this perspective of Health Education, becomes responsible for training professionals who establish a reciprocal relationship with society (ALMEIDA, 2003; CECCIM, FEUERWEKER, 2004a; HADDAD et al., 2006).

Through the SUS and the Family Health Strategy (ESF), some specific ways of teaching and learning must be prioritized. The ESF is fundamental to the implementation of the Basic Care Policy (BRASIL, 2006), as it focuses on the family, where health is seen not only as the absence of disease, but also taking into account factors such as food, housing, basic sanitation, the environment, work, income, education, transport, leisure and access to essential goods and services (BRASIL, 1990). The ESF prioritizes teamwork, shared responsibility in the planning and execution of support, as well as the *interdisciplinarity* and *comprehensiveness* that must be present in this support (ROSA, LABATE, 2005).

In the context of ESF teaching, the preceptor is a professional who is not from academia but from the service, with higher education in the health area, and has the role of narrowing the gap between theory and practice in the training of students. The role of this professional is to guide, support, teach and share experiences that improve the student's skills (BOTTI, REGO, 2008). It is hoped that the relationship between the preceptor and the student will be horizontal, that the act of thinking and building hypotheses will be encouraged and that the student will discover, in this relationship, the importance of collective work (BARRETO et al., 2011).

The preceptor should be primarily concerned with clinical competence and the teaching-learning aspects of professional development, as well as encouraging the acquisition of skills and competences for students in the practice settings where they are located. It is also up to the preceptor to create the necessary conditions for changes to be implemented satisfactorily during the students' training process (BOTTI, REGO, 2008).

From this perspective, one of the main challenges facing higher education in Brazil is to overcome concepts linked only to technical and biological knowledge, which favors the development of interdisciplinary and comprehensive care (FEUERWERKER, 2003; SMEKE, OLIVEIRA, 2001; FURTADO, 2009).

To this end, interdisciplinarity enables the training of professionals who have a minimum chance of working together and creating the conditions for more integrated care for SUS users (CARDOSO et al., 2007). It is necessary to transform health concepts and practices that guide the process of academic and professional training in health (GONZALEZ, ALMEIDA, 2010; CECCIM, FEUERWEKER, 2004b).

Concomitant with the fragmentation and excessive specialization of knowledge, the result of technological advances and the isolation of disciplines, interdisciplinarity has been at the center of discussions about the development of science and health practices (MATOS, PIRES, CAMPOS, 2009).

In this context, it became feasible to ask the question of this research: How are the preceptors of the family health units of the II Sanitary District of Maceio acting in terms of interdisciplinarity?

3.2 Methodology

This study, carried out in the field of health teaching, was a descriptive study with a qualitative approach. The research was carried out in the 2nd Health District (HD) of the Municipality of Maceio-AL, which is currently divided into seven HDs, geographical areas that are organized on a territorial basis with similar epidemiological and social characteristics.

This research allowed us to get closer to the central object of study - *interdisciplinarity* - through the information gathered during the research process.

The objective of this study was to analyze how interdisciplinarity is used by preceptors in the ESF health support units in the 2nd District of Maceio. And more specifically: to find out about the preceptors' practices related to interdisciplinarity; to understand the preceptors' academic/professional training in interdisciplinarity; to analyze the benefits of interdisciplinary practices in the students' teaching-learning process; to propose suggestions to the Higher Education Institution and the Municipal Health Department regarding interdisciplinary practice.

The choice of data collection instrument was based on a theoretical study of the object of study. We opted for the "open-ended or in-depth interview" data collection instrument (Minayo, Gomes, 2011, p. 64), with guiding questions, which allowed the interviewer to broadly explore the desired issues.

After the theoretical deepening phase and the preparation of the data collection instrument, the subjects were recruited. For this purpose, the following inclusion criteria were used: to be an ESF preceptor at one of the units that make up the 2nd HD of Maceio; to be a health professional with higher education; to be receiving students from higher education institutions during the research period. Failure to meet any of the criteria was considered the only exclusion criterion. In this way, four of the five ESF teams in this district were included in the study.

According to the inclusion criteria, all the subjects agreed to take part in this study after signing the Free and Informed Consent Form. There were a total of nine subjects, from four ESFs in the 2nd HD of the municipality of Maceio.

The universe of subjects is presented in Tables 1 and 2 (see below), containing personal identification data (characterization of the research subjects) and complementary data on professional practice.

Table 1 - Characterization of the participants in the study research

Name	Age	Gener	Formapao Academics - Graduation	Year completed	Complementary Training
Subject 1	45	F	Medicine	1991	Residency in Pediatrics; Clinical Medicine Residency
Subject 2	41	F	Physiotherapy	1993	Masters in Public Health

Subject 3	44	M	Medicine	1991	Residency in General Surgery and Urology; Specialization in Family Health
Subject 4	58	M	Medicine	1978	Residency in Internal Medicine
Subject 5	54	F	Nursing	1978	Master in Health Sciences
Subject 6	35	F	Social Services	2000	Postgraduate course in Management and Social Control of Public Policies
Subject 7	54	F	Nursing	1979	Specialization in Family Health; Urgency-Emergency Specialization
Subject 8	40	F	Nursing	1991	Specialization in Hospital Administration; Specialization in Auditing; Specialization in Urgency-Emergency
Subject 9	44	F	Medicine	1995	Specialization in Pediatrics

Source: Author, 2013.

Table 2 - Additional data on professional practice

Name	Have you participated in any training for the position of preceptor (yes/no) / Institution that offered it	Training characteristics (theoretical, practical, theoretical-practical)	Do you teach at a Higher Education Institution - HEI (yes/no) / Institution	Other workplaces
Subject 1	No	-	No	---

Subject 2	No	-	Yes/ Public HEI	Hospital Private, HEI Public and HEI Private
Subject 3	No	-	No	Public Hospital
Subject 4	No	-	Yes/Public HEI	Private practice
Subject 5	No	-	Yes/ IES Private	Public HEI and Private HEI
Subject 6	Yes/ Maceio Municipal Health Department	Theoretical	No	---
Subject 7	No	-	No	---
Subject 8	No	-	No	---
Subject 9	Yes/ Sirio Libanes Hospital	Theory and practice	No	Public hospital and private practice

Source: ora, 2013.

To analyze the data, we chose Thematic Analysis, which uses the "theme" (Bardin, 1979, p. 111) as its central concept and can be graphically presented through a message; this can be a word, a sentence or a summary (Minayo, Gomes, 2011, p.86). And to analyze the content of these messages, we used Registration Units (UR) (Minayo, Gomes, 2011, p.87).

All the interview recordings were transcribed in full. This material was then thoroughly read in order to appropriate the content, following the model for treatment, compilation and analysis, as recommended by the literature (Bardin, 1979; Minayo, Gomes, 2011). In order to interpret the data, the research results were compared with the theoretical framework on Interdisciplinarity, ESF, Health Teaching, in the search for coherent, singular or contradictory content.

After *analyzing the content of* the answers described by the participants, the common reports and the proximity to the object of this study, the Registration Units (UR) were named as follows:

UR 1. activities you carry out in your day-to-day work at the ESF

UR 2 Experience in daily professional practice

UR 3 Meaning of Interdisciplinarity

UR 4. academic/professional training in interdisciplinary practice

UR 5. benefits of interdisciplinary practices in the students' teaching-learning process

UR 6. suggestions for improving interdisciplinary practice

3.3 Results and Discussion

In the first UR (UR1), which refers to the *activities you carry out in your day-to-day work at the ESF,* most of the speeches focused on curative care, and none of the reports dealt with teamwork, or with these health teams prioritizing health prevention and promotion. It should be noted that these preventive and promotive educational supports, as well as being recommended by the ESF, also enable the integration of the different professional categories present in the health teams and should be part of the daily work of these ESF teams.

Subject 2. As we have a pent-up demand, home care is also provided.

Subject 3. Here at the ESF, we work with consultations aimed at covering the various programs that are part of the ESF, including consultations with hypertensive patients, diabetics, women's health [...].

Subject 6. On a day-to-day basis, we provide individual care; during these appointments, I also make referrals.

Subject 7. I do the strategy programs, right? Women's health, prenatal care, growth- development, such as home visits.

Subject 8. I provide prenatal care, growth and development, childcare, hypertension, diabetes, family planning, cytology, visits and talks.

Saupe et al. (2005), in their research, state that interdisciplinarity is one of the elements, or one of the paths, that makes it possible to get closer to a Comprehensive Health Care practice.

And comprehensiveness must be linked to the need to change a fragmented and disjointed way of acting in health, as seen in UR1. In order to change this disjointed and individualistic practice, the ESF has emerged as an action tool of the SUS, possibly effective in operationalizing health practice with an interdisciplinary vision. And these interdisciplinary practices, in the teaching sphere, are fundamental for health training.

It was observed, then, that interdisciplinary actions, following the guiding principles of the SUS, such as integrality, present challenges in health education. One of these challenges is to offer a counterbalance to the influence of the fragmented model of work organization, in which each professional carries out parts of the work without integration with the other areas involved.

Thus, in their study, Garcia et al. (2007) argue that, in the National Curriculum Guidelines, health is considered an interdisciplinary area, since its object, which would be the human health-disease process, involves social relations, biology and emotional expressions. Albuquerque and Stotz (2004), in turn, point to the importance of collective actions, valuing the knowledge of others. It is thus understood that knowledge is a process of shared construction, which provides a greater understanding of interdisciplinary actions in health.

UR2 deals with *experience in daily professional practice.* The research participants provided data on interpersonal relationships between team members. The subjects justified the fact that they did not prioritize interdisciplinary activities due to the high demand from the population for individual care, i.e. specialized care. The results of this UR showed that the professionals interviewed do not experience interdisciplinary health actions in their respective ESF teams.

Subject 1: I don't have any problems with the team.

Subject 3: Every daily work situation that I have, I'm the one who does the planning, within the needs that we find at work. [...] the relationship with the other professionals, nursing technicians, nurses and everything is within the standard of respect for their space. That's it.

Subject 4. Sometimes I even find myself doing traditional medicine, because the anxiety of the population is the medical consultation, the demand, and they want us to attend and more and more [...] we've been trying to work on the team, we've even been trying to work on what a family health team would be, but the need is so great, the suffering is so great!

Subject 7. But I think I experience the difficulties in my day-to-day work. A lot of difficulties, especially in getting along with other professionals. We get on well, but we each do our own thing, without invading the other's space.

Subject 9: And with my team, I have a good relationship, you know? With the nurse in my team, with the health workers, right?

The results of this research showed that, within professional practice, which values teamwork, the health professionals who were the subjects of this study do not prioritize interaction between the different disciplines, especially when this communication is aimed at interdisciplinary health practices. Most of the time, this was justified by the subjects as a lack of time for dialogue. This lack of time may suggest an obstacle to the interaction of disciplines, since they need mutual cooperation for interdisciplinary actions to take place in a concrete way.

According to Japiassu (1976, p.123), this communication takes place through interdisciplinary methodology, which means, first and foremost, "talking about operating and cooperating disciplines". This emphasizes the importance of dialogue between the different professional categories for interdisciplinary practice to take place.

As Peduzzi (1998) points out, it is essential to value spaces for reflection among health workers as spaces for exchange, interaction and communication. In this way, the subjects reported the need to reorganize the work in the ESF so that there is finally the possibility of interaction between the professional categories in health.

In UR3, which deals with the *Meaning of Interdisciplinarity*, there was a lack of knowledge of the concept of *interdisciplinarity.* Some professionals were confused with *multidisciplinarity* and some even came close to the meaning of interdisciplinarity. However, in this case, interdisciplinarity is seen as something theoretical only, with no connection to interdisciplinary practice.

Subject 1. Inter what? What do you want to know? [...] working with other professionals? [...] we work together.

Subject 3 (laughs) Interdisciplinarity... I understand it like this, and... interdisciplinarity... Let me see... I understand that interdisciplinarity would be a... A range of professionals working on different activities, but complementing each other. We doctors [...]. We want things to be immediate,

But things don't work immediately. So we suffer a lot in this interdisciplinary process.

Subject 4: But I haven't yet managed, perhaps because of the dynamics of the training process, to train medical students in this interdisciplinary way. There is a relationship between the categories, but I haven't yet managed to bring it together, to make medical students experience it in practice, even though they feel that we do.

Subject 6. We do a single piece of work, but it's broken down in such a way that the user understands what we're talking about.

Subject 7: Interdisciplinarity? Interdisciplinarity? I think it's when there's teamwork, isn't it? These concepts are very complicated! Everyone says it's one thing. But I think it's when you manage to work together, with several professionals, right?

Subject 8: I think it's a combination of various professions... the doctor, the nurse, the dentist. Everyone together. Is that it? I'm not sure. [...] Then we work together.

Subject 9: You do your bit, but so what? There are things you need, right? Contact with others.

In his study, Trentin (2010) also pointed out that the subjects had great difficulty in conceptualizing interdisciplinarity when it was related to practice, with a tendency towards multidisciplinarity. In multidisciplinary organizations, there are different professional categories that don't necessarily talk to each other. According to Japiassu (1976), for interdisciplinarity to happen, there must be interaction between disciplines around a common goal, in the construction of new knowledge.

Other issues also arose in UR3, such as the fact that most of the professionals showed that they knew that working in an interdisciplinary way was essential in the ESF and, as preceptors, present in the students' training, they recognized that they were responsible for transmitting interdisciplinary practice in the ESF to the students. However, they identified the limitations of their academic training with regard to the theory and practice of interdisciplinarity.

In their research, Ronzani and Stralen (2003) state that the practice of professionals in the ESF is still based on super-specialized training and the isolation of professional categories. This isolation of disciplines can be seen in the speech fragments of the subjects of this study, especially when one observes a re-focusing of health support only on curative and individual practices and a distancing from health promotion and disease prevention support, which are essential in the ESF and essential for an understanding of interdisciplinarity.

It can be seen that the limitations of the preceptor's academic training refer to their training. This professional needs to be recognized for his role as the protagonist of the students' curricular practices with regard to Interdisciplinarity.

To this end, Moretti-Pires (2009) suggests that, insofar as health professionals and future professionals learn only the technical aspects of their profession and do not understand how to articulate with other professional categories, university training alone will not enable interdisciplinary action.

In this way, it is believed that the deepening of scientific knowledge and technical advances alone are not enough to cover the area of health. Thus, interdisciplinarity is seen as a facilitator in building a broader vision, based on the integration of different professional categories and with the aim of developing new knowledge.

In UR4, which dealt with *academic/professional training with regard to interdisciplinary practice,* the majority of subjects did not say that they had known or experienced interdisciplinarity during their academic training. In professional training, the search for knowledge of interdisciplinarity proved to be an individual initiative.

Subject 1 At the time, it wasn't even talked about. I come from a totally different background to today.

Subject 4: My training [...] was medicine and medicine with illness in mind. Just medicine. Although the course said that it was supposed to train general practitioners and blah-blah-blah, in practice it wasn't, it wasn't because we only saw subjects and the subjects talked about the diseases of each subject.

Subject 5: But in my training there wasn't any, and we don't see this practice, neither in the faculties, nor in the service, of trying to adjust, right?

Subject 7: I didn't have anything in my degree, not that I can remember. It was just nursing with nursing. That's it. In the postgraduate course I did, it was all theory, I didn't have anything practical to do with the team, even in the specialization I did with other professional categories, it was everyone doing their own thing, talking about their own area.

Subject 8: I've never had anything like that. Neither during my undergraduate or postgraduate studies. I don't think I really know what interdisciplinarity is.

These professionals reported working as part of a team, but showed difficulty in carrying out this practice within the ESF and passing on this interdisciplinary training to students. The majority of the preceptors in this study were unaware of the theory/practice of interdisciplinarity, bringing it closer to other concepts, such as multidisciplinarity and disciplinarity. Thus, these subjects showed an interest in learning about interdisciplinarity, since it seems to be indispensable for professional practice in the ESF and essential in the training of students.

Favarao and Araujo (2004) argue that today's society requires universities not only to train academics for future qualifications in traditional specializations, but also to train them to develop their skills and abilities in the light of new knowledge that is being produced and which requires a new type of professional, without dissociating theory from practice. This new knowledge mainly concerns the ability to work from an interdisciplinary perspective and to be aware of the contributions of other professional categories.

Knowledge of other professions allows us to broaden our view of the field of health and, consequently, the integrated construction of new knowledge. This knowledge, in turn, is developed through the intersection of different professional categories. This integration of disciplines/professions can only be understood more concretely when interdisciplinary theory and practice are linked. In this way, the practice setting, during the students' academic training, is the privileged place to understand interdisciplinarity, especially when this setting is the ESF, one of the fields where the principles and guidelines of the SUS are put into practice.

Therefore, it is necessary to provide spaces for interaction in practice settings, and it is also necessary for the professional preceptor to be made aware of their leading role in the curricular practices of students with regard to interdisciplinarity (SAUPE et al, 2005).

The preceptor, in this space of service and academic training, must become one of the main facilitators of interdisciplinary practice. This benefits both the population assisted through integrated health support and the training of students. In addition, the student's training must also be seen as integral by the training institution.

This comprehensive training facilitates the building of a cooperative relationship between teacher/preceptor and student. This, in turn, is believed to open the way to recognizing the importance of interaction with other areas of academic training. According to Morin (2001, p.13), "An education can only be viable if it is an integral education of the human being. An education that addresses the open totality of the human being and not just one of its components".

In UR5, which dealt with the *benefits of interdisciplinary practices in the teaching-learning process of students,* the subjects recognized that interdisciplinarity is important and can make a difference in the training of future professionals for the SUS, even though the previous URs showed that the subjects themselves do not practice and/or are unaware of interdisciplinarity.

Subject 1: Yes, there is. Everyone has to see each other's professional value, right?

Subject 3. From the point of view of colleagues from other specialties, other professions, they see us as adversaries, but we're not anyone's adversaries, we just want things to be done according to what should be done. So, for me, I'm not opposed, as long as my competence isn't usurped, it isn't invaded.

Subject 4. I think so, and one of the things I always say and try to do is that the doctor is not the all-powerful master of a team and that each professional has their importance in what we set out to do.

Subject 6: It's very, very important. We have to know the following: we are [...] a team. Ideally, everyone should think like that [...] this is very important for the student's education, so that they also learn. I think medicine is very individualistic, right?

Subject 7: [...] working as a team, seeing what each other is doing. There's resistance from the medical profession too. Especially from students... I think it must be the training. Then there are these barriers that prevent it.

Subject 8. Yes, I think there should be benefits, right? Working together with the agents, with the dentist, at least making the visits, should already be a big gain. It's an impact for them to get out into the community, to communicate with the other professionals.

Subject 9: My medical students don't take part in interdisciplinary support, unfortunately. If they did, they'd benefit, wouldn't they?

The professionals seem to show that the main benefit of interdisciplinarity in the training of students is linked only to interpersonal relationships. It is believed that the benefits go beyond this relationship, as it enables the integrated construction of health actions and the recognition of other professional categories in the construction of a new method/object. In this way, interdisciplinarity can be seen as an alternative to the excessive fragmentation of knowledge and help to develop new knowledge (PAVIANE, 2003).

Another issue that was observed in the results of this study was the resistance of the medical profession to possible work interdisciplinary. This was mainly brought up by medical and nursing professionals. The medical professionals themselves reported the difficulty of working with their professional category. They pointed to some issues to justify this resistance, such as: poor academic/professional training with regard to interdisciplinarity; the academic focus on technical-curative practices; and excessive demand for outpatient care in health units.

In their research, Garcia et al. (2007) concluded that the centrality of the biomedical model, with its focus on technical-curative practices, makes it difficult to bring the different professional categories closer together, maintaining the perspective of 'help' between professionals and referring to "prejudice" and "arrogance". The centrality of the biomedical model is one of the reasons why it is difficult to achieve more integrated and better quality health action, both from the perspective of those who carry it out and those who benefit from it (MATOS, PIRES, CAMPOS, 2009; MORETTI-PIRES, 2009). Interdisciplinary action can also provide an alternative form of differentiated training, based on a broad view of health problems and the understanding that knowledge and interdisciplinary action are not mutually exclusive, but intersect.

The last Registration Unit (UR6), which dealt with *Suggestions for improving interdisciplinary practice,* showed that professionals need training in interdisciplinarity from a theoretical-practical perspective. Training was suggested by the preceptors to be an initiative of the Higher Education Institution responsible for the students in the practice settings and also of the Municipal Health Department, which is responsible for the health services, such as the ESF.

The preceptors recognized that their academic and professional training was deficient in terms of interdisciplinary theory and practice. They revealed the need they felt to improve their support, both to improve health services and to collaborate more effectively in the academic training of students, in terms of interdisciplinarity.

Subject 2. Okay, a suggestion: I think what would be interesting would be training for the staff, right? Training focused on interdisciplinarity. It's never been done. How can it be passed on to the students? There has to be training. [...] Someone with experience should do this, right? Someone from the municipality or the university, someone who has practiced.

Subject 3. Something interdisciplinary. I don't know what idea I'd give. I don't know what the practices are. I don't understand. I don't know how this situation is done, you know? I think that, perhaps, we need the gaze of the academy and the gaze of the secretariat to train us in this and to receive these students, to be able to teach them, right?

Subject 5: And in relation to interdisciplinary practice, something to standardize interdisciplinary and health education practices. For that to happen, the university would have to offer something for the preceptors, training on this to standardize it for us, to help train the kids, right? Something that would be common to everyone.

Subject 6: The service needs to be visited by the university. The university could train the preceptors in this interdisciplinary work, but they don't even know what we do in the service with their students, do they?

Subject 7: We've never had anything about interdisciplinarity. Couldn't the university train us? Take us there? Do something with everyone. And the municipal health department, too, only thinks about the disease, so we teach the students what we've learned, right?

Subject 8. I think what's missing is the university here with us, closer to us, seeing our work, as well as the municipal office. That's not what our training was for. How are we going to help the students in this sense? They need to come and decipher the question of interdisciplinarity. Meet, discuss and chew. I might think that's not what it really means. I need to know, don't I? And once I've opened up the range of possibilities for us, I can find out how to pass them on to the students.

Suggestions for training in interdisciplinary theory and practice should be considered, given that the ESF is a proposal to change the work process in primary care and is an open field for the teaching-learning process of future health professionals, as advocated by the laws governing the SUS.

The results of this research showed, as in the study by More et al. (2004), that the interaction between the members of a health team raises several questions about the attitude of these professionals, especially with regard to common support. For these supports to be effective, it is necessary to train the professionals involved in the health teams to develop and work with interdisciplinary practices.

For training to take place, there needs to be recognition of its necessity on the part of the professionals directly involved in integrated support for health teams, as well as on the part of the institutions that train and maintain health services. Loch-Neckel, et al. (2009) suggest that interdisciplinary training is needed to recognize interdisciplinary work and its importance for the training of future health professionals for the SUS.

Thus, there needs to be a dialog between the Higher Education Institution, the Municipal Health Department and the practice settings that enable training, such as the ESF, represented by the preceptor professionals. These professionals need to be permanently trained both for the preceptorship function, since they are present in the students' academic training, and for the health services, such as the ESF.

This SUS strategy (ESF) needs professionals who are able to work in a shared way, by accepting other knowledge. For this integrated practice to take place, it is necessary to go beyond technical-scientific knowledge. In addition to an academic education focused on interdisciplinarity, it is necessary to train the professionals who are working in the service and who have already passed through the academy and have not had this broader health education. What is needed is permanent training that integrates the professional categories, without segregation, in search of interdisciplinarity.

3.4 Final considerations

The data pointed to a lack of awareness of interdisciplinarity on the part of the professional preceptors in this study, both in terms of theory and interdisciplinary practice. This lack of knowledge was due to the fact that the subjects did not have an academic education focused on interdisciplinarity, nor did they have any training in interdisciplinary practice or theory during their experiences in the professional field.

The preceptors recognized the importance of interdisciplinarity for the training of future professionals, but also that they were not prepared to pass on knowledge to students from an interdisciplinary perspective, since they were not trained with a broader view of the concept of health.

As a suggestion for improving work in the ESF and as assets in the training of future professionals for the SUS, the preceptors suggested training on the subject of interdisciplinarity. It was suggested that this training be coordinated by the SMS and the higher education institution responsible for the students in the ESF practice settings.

The conclusions drawn from this research do not exhaust the subject in question. By studying how interdisciplinarity and instrumentalized by preceptors in the ESF, the aim was to demonstrate the importance of practice and theory interdisciplinarity in working relationships and in health training for the SUS. But other influences and aspects can and should be considered in the study of interdisciplinarity. Therefore, this research points to new and productive studies.

REFERENCES

ALBUQUERQUE, P. C.; STOTZ, E. N. Popular education in basic health care in the municipality: in search of integrality. **Interface - Comunicação, Saude, Educagao**, Botucatu, v.8, n.15, mar./ago. p.259-74, 2004.

ALMEIDA, M. et al. (Org.). Diretrizes curriculares nacionais para os cursos universitárias da área da saúde. Londrina: Rede Unida; 2003.

BARDIN, L. **Content analysis**. Lisbon: Edigoes 70, 1976.

BARRETO, V. H. et al. Role of the primary health care preceptor in undergraduate and postgraduate training at the Federal University of Pernambuco - a Term of Reference. **Rev. Bras. Educ. Med.**, v. 35, n. 4, p. 578-583, 2011.

BOTTI, S.; REGO, S. Preceptor, supervisor, tutor and mentor: what are their roles? **Rev. Bras. Educ. Med**. v. 32. n. 3, p. 363-373, 2008.

BRAZIL. Law no. 8.080, of September 19, 1990. Provides on the conditions for the promotion, protection and recovery of health, the organization and operation of the corresponding services and other measures. **Diario Oficial [da] Republica Federativa do** Brasil, Poder Legislativo, Brasilia, DF, September 20, 1990, Section 1, p. 18055.

. Ordinance No. 648/GM, of March 28, 2006. National Primary Care Policy. Disposes of the guidelines and norms for the organization of Primary Care. **Diario Oficial [da] Republica Federativa do** Brasil, Brasilia, DF, March 28, 2006. Section 1, p 71.

. Ministry of Education. CNE/CNS Resolution No. 4 of February 19, 2002. Institutes National Curricular Guidelines for the Physiotherapy Degree Course. **Diario Oficial [da] Republica Federativa do** Brasil, Brasilia, DF, 4 mar. 2002a. Sepao 1, p. 11.

. CNE/CNS Resolution No. 6 of February 19, 2002. Institutes National Curricular Guidelines for the Degree Course in Occupational Therapy. **Diario Oficial [da] Republica Federativa do** Brasil, Brasilia, DF, 4 mar. 2002b. Section 1, p. 12.

. CNE/CES Resolution No. 4 of November 7, 2001. Establishes National Curricular Guidelines for the Undergraduate Degree in Medicine. **Diario Oficial [da] Republica Federativa do Brasil**, Brasilia, DF, de 9 nov. 2001a. Section 1, p. 38.

. CNE/CES Resolution No. 3 of November 7, 2001. Institutes National Curricular Guidelines for Undergraduate Nursing Courses. **Diario Oficial [da] Republica Federativa do Brasil**, Brasilia, DF, 9 nov. 2001b. Section 1, p. 37.

CARDOSO, J. P. et al. Formapao Interdisciplinar: Efetivando Propostas de Promopao da Saude no SUS. **Rev. Bras. em Promopao da Saude**, Fortaleza, v. 20. n. 4, p. 252-258, 2007.

CECCIM, R.B.; FEUERWEKER, L. C. M. The quadrilateral of health training: teaching, management, care and social control.
Physis: Rev. Saude Coletiva, Rio de Janeiro, v.14, n.1, jan./jun., p. 41-65, 2004a.

;. Changes in the graduation of health professions under the axis of integrality. **Cad. Saude Publica**, Rio de Janeiro, v.20, n.5, Sept./Oct., p. 1400-10, 2004b.

FAVARAO, N. R. L; ARAUJO, C. S. A. The importance of interdisciplinarity in higher education. **Educere**, Umuarama, v. 4, n. 2, Jul./Dec. p.103-115, 2004.

FEUERWERKER, L. C. M. **Beyond the discourse of change in medical education**: processes and results. Sao Paulo: Hucitec, 2002.

. Education of health professionals today: problems, challenges, perspectives and the proposals of the Ministry of Health. **Revista da ABENO**, Brasilia, DF, v. 3, n. 1, p. 24-27, 2003.

FURTADO, J.P. Institutional arrangements and clinic management: principles of interdisciplinarity and interprofessionality. **Cad. Bras. Saude Mental**, v. 1, n. 1, jan./abr. 2009.

GARCIA, M. L. A. et al. Interdisciplinarity necessary for medical education. **Rev. Bras. Educ. Med.**, v. 31, n.2, p. 147 - 155; 2007.

GARCIA, M. L. A. et al. Interdisciplinarity and Integrality in Health Teaching. **Rev. Cienc. Med.**, Campinas, v. 15, n. 6, p. 473-485, Nov./Dec. 2006.

GATTAS, M.L.G. **Interdisciplinaridade**: formapao e apao na área de saude. Ribeirao Preto: Holos, 2006.

GUEDES, L. E.; FERREIRA JUNIOR, M. Disciplinary relationships in a teaching and research center in health promotion and disease prevention practices. **Rev. Saude Sociedade**, Sao Paulo, v. 19, n. 2, p.260-272, 2010.

GONZALEZ, A. D.; ALMEIDA, M. J. Integrality of health: guiding changes in the training of new professionals. **Cienc. Saude Colet.**, v. 15, n. 3, p. 757-62, 2010.

HADDAD, A.E, et al. (Org.). **The trajectory of undergraduate health courses** 1991-2004. Brasilia, DF: INEP, 2006.

JAPIASSU, H. **Interdisciplinaridade e patologia do saber.** Rio de Janeiro: Imago, 1976.

LINARD, A. G.; CASTRO, M. M.; CRUZ, A. K. L. Comprehensive care as understood by family health strategy professionals. **Rev. Gaucha Enferm.**, Porto Alegre, v. 32, n. 3, p. 546-53, 2011.

LOCH-NECKEL, G. et al. Challenges for interdisciplinary action in primary care: implications for the composition of family health teams. **Cienc. Saude Colet.**, v. 14, n. 1, p. 1463-1472, 2009.

MATOS, E; PIRES, D. E. P; CAMPOS, G. W. S. Working relationships in interdisciplinary teams: contributions to the constitution of new forms of health work organization. **Rev. Bras. Enferm.**, Brasilia, DF, v. 62, n. 6, nov./dez. p.863-9, 2009.

MATTOS, R. A. The meanings of comprehensiveness: some reflections on values that deserve to be defended. In: PINHEIRO, R.; MATTOS, R. (Org.). **Os sentidos da integralidade na atenpao e no cuidado em saude**. 4. ed. Rio de Janeiro: Cepesc/ IMS/Uerj/Abrasco, 2005.

MINAYO, M. C. S.; GOMES, S. F. D. **Pesquisa social**: teoria, metodo e criatividade. 30. ed. Petropolis: Vozes, 2011.

MORE, C. et al. The social representations of the psychologist among residents of the family health program and the importance of interdisciplinarity. **Rev. Psicologia Hospitalar**, v. 1, n. 1, p. 59-75, 2004.

MORIN, E. A. **Cabepa bem-feita**: repensar a reformar o pensamento. Translated by Eloa Jacobina. 5. ed. Rio de Janeiro: Bertrand Brasil, 2001.

MORETTI-PIRES, R. O. Complexidade em Saude da Familia e formapao do futuro profissional de saude. **Interface - Comunicapao, Saude, Educapao**, Botucatu, v. 13, n. 30, jul./set. p. 153-66, 2009.

PAVIANE, J. Disciplinarity and interdisciplinarity. In: INTERNATIONAL SEMINAR INTERDISCIPLINARITY, HUMANISM, 1., 2003. Porto. **Proceedings**... Porto: University of Porto, November 12-14, 2003.

PEDUZZI, M. **Multiprofessional health team**: the interface between work and interaction. 1998. Thesis (Doctorate in Collective Health) - State University of Campinas. Campinas, 1998.

ROSA, W. A. G; LABATE, R. C. Family Health Program: the construction of a new care model. **Rev. Latino Americana de Enfermagem**. Sao Paulo, v. 13, n. 6, p.1027-34, 2005.

RONZANI, T. M; STRALEN, C. J. V. Dificuldades de Implantapao do Programa de Saude da Familia como estrategia de reforma do sistema de saude brasileiro. **Revista APS**, v. 6, n. 2, jul./dez. p.99-107, 2003.

SAUPE, R. et al. Competence of health professionals for interdisciplinary work. **Interface - Comunicapao, Saude, Educapao, Botucatu**, v. 9, n. 18, set./dez., p.521-36, 2005.

SMEKE, E. L. M.; OLIVEIRA, N. L. S. Health education and conceptions of the subject. In: VASCONCELOS, E. M. et al. **A saude nas palavras e nos gestos**: reflexoes da rede educapao popular e saude. Sao Paulo: HUCITEC, 2001. p.115-136.

TRETIN, V. R. M. **Interdisciplinary practices in training processes in health services**. 2010. Monograph (Specialization in Pedagogical Practices for Education in Health Services) - Federal University of Rio Grande do Sul. Porto Alegre, 2010.

4 INTERVENTION PROJECT

Interdisciplinarity in Health Education: Reframing collective actions through a shared and integrated vision

4.1 Introduction

One of the National Constitution's guidelines for health actions and services, when constituted as a single system, is comprehensive care, i.e. the integrality of care as a guiding constitutional principle for the formulation of health policies (BRASIL, 1990). This comprehensiveness is present in the guidelines of the Unified Health System (SUS): decentralization; comprehensive care; and community participation. In this way, the SUS has taken on an active role in discussing and reorienting strategies and ways of caring for, treating and monitoring individual and collective health. This reinforces the need to train professionals to act in accordance with this new health policy (CECCIM, FEUERWERKER, 2004).

The Family Health Strategy (ESF) is one of the most effective instruments for operationalizing the National Primary Care Policy (BRASIL, 2006). It is a fundamental strategy at the primary care level, as it prioritizes teamwork, shared responsibility in the planning and execution of actions, as well as interdisciplinarity and comprehensiveness (ROSA, LABATE, 2005).

The ESF is also an open practice scenario for the teaching-learning process of students from the various health and humanities courses, since it is a field that enables the construction of a broader view of health, not just as the absence of disease, but taking into account factors such as nutrition, housing, basic sanitation, the environment, work, income, education, transport, leisure and access to essential goods and services (BRASIL, 1990), thus contributing to a more humanistic, interdisciplinary education, with a view to improving the quality of life of the population assisted.

However, even though the ESF is a field that enables differentiated training in line with the new Curricular Guidelines for Undergraduate Health Courses, it requires attention for the training and qualification of its professionals, who, in most cases, as well as carrying out their duties within the ESF, participate in the training of students at Higher Education Institutions (HEIs), acting as preceptors.

The preceptor is a professional who is not from the academy but from the service, with higher education in the health area and has the important role of narrowing the gap between theory and practice in the training of students. This professional has the following functions: to guide, support, teach and share experiences that improve the student's skills (BOTTI, REGO, 2008). It is hoped that the relationship between the preceptor and the student will be horizontal, that the act of thinking and building hypotheses will be encouraged and that the student will discover, in this relationship, the importance of collective work (BARRETO et al., 2011).

The preceptor is mainly concerned with clinical competence or the teaching-learning aspects of professional development, as well as promoting the acquisition of skills and competences for students in the practice settings where they are located. It is up to the preceptor to create the necessary conditions for changes to be implemented satisfactorily during the students' training process (BOTTI, REGO, 2008).

The ESF preceptor has a very relevant differential, which is that he or she is in a field that in itself enables a broader view of health, through shared, collective and integrated practices. However, it can be seen that in most ESF practice scenarios, students are unable to put these aforementioned supports into practice, reproducing technical-curative supports. These approaches also fail to comply with the SUS/FHS guidelines, whose main possibility for intervention is interdisciplinary practice, inducing students to move away from traditional academic positions towards new perspectives and new paths in health teaching.

In this context, the research entitled: "Interdisciplinarity in Health Teaching: the view of the preceptor in the Family Health Strategy" was carried out, with the main objective of "Analyzing how interdisciplinarity is used by preceptors in the health supports of the Family Health Units of the II Sanitary District of Maceio". This research is part of a professional master's thesis from the Health Teaching Program at the Faculty of Medicine (FAMED) of the Federal University of Alagoas (UFAL).

Based on the planning, execution, theoretical deepening and discussion of the results, this research suggests a relevant and significant demand from the subjects - ESF preceptors from the II Sanitary District of Maceio - for theoretical and practical training in relation to the theme of "Interdisciplinarity", carried out by the HEI in partnership with the Municipal Health Department (SMS) of Maceio, with the proposal of bringing the HEI closer to the practice scenarios of its students. This suggestion of training on the theme of interdisciplinarity should be considered, given that the ESF is a proposal to change the work process in primary care, and is an open field for the teaching-learning process of future health professionals, as advocated by the laws governing the SUS.

3.1.1 Characterization of the research site "Interdisciplinarity in Health Teaching: the preceptor's view of the Family Health Strategy"

The Municipality of Maceio-AL is divided into 7 (seven) Health Districts, which comprise geographical areas that are organized on a territorial basis with similar epidemiological and social characteristics. The research took place in the II Sanitary District of Maceio, which is part of the Health Network of this District: 1 (one) Dental Module; 2 (two) Health Centers; and 2 (two) Health Centers.

Medical Specialties (PAM Breda and PAM Dique Estrada); 1 (one) Health Unit that attends to spontaneous demand (Unidade de Saude Rolland Simon); and 5 (five) Family Health Units - USF (Unidade de Saude da Familia Helvio Auto (Rua Riachuelo, 20, Trapiche), Unidade de Saude da Familia Jardim Sao Francisco (Rua Sao Francisco, 02, Brejal), Unidade de Saude da Familia Virgem dos Pobres (Av. Senador Rui Palmeira, s/n, Dique Estrada), Tarcisio Palmeira Family Health Unit (Rua Alipio Barbosa, s/n, Pontal da Barra), Professor Durval Cortez Family Health Unit (Rua Joao Ulisses Marques, s/n, Prado). The latter is the most recent USF in this district, and at the time of the survey the professionals were not receiving students from the Higher Education Institutes (HEIs); for this reason, this unit was not included in the survey. Thus, 4 (four) USFs that make up the Health Network of this District were included.

The II Sanitary District of Maceio is characterized by being a differentiated region, especially in physical and cultural terms. A large part of this district lies between the sea and the lagoon, favoring mainly characteristic work activities such as fishing and handicrafts.

The HEI Universidade Estadual de Ciencias da Saude de Alagoas - UNCISAL is located in this district. It has 5 (five) bachelor's degrees in the health area (Nursing, Physiotherapy, Speech Therapy, Medicine and Occupational Therapy) and 4 (four) technological degrees (Technology in Systems Analysis and Development, Technology in Management Processes, Technology in Radiology, Technology in Biomedical Systems). All the units are undergoing a process of reorganization of the Family Health Strategy, mainly because they are, for the most part, practice scenarios for the HEI present in this Health District.

Thus, after a thorough theoretical study, an approach to the research topic and the results of the research, this project was drawn up with the aim of offering a response to the subjects of the study, the HEI and the SMS, as a form of research product. This project will initially be sent to UNCISAL's Dean of Education and Graduation (PROEG). It is hoped that this Pro-Rectory will begin to mobilize this intervention project in partnership with the SMS. This could contribute to the teaching-learning process for students and to the training of professional preceptors in the service, with regard to interdisciplinarity in health teaching, more specifically in ESF practice settings.

4.2 Target audience

Higher education health professionals who are part of the Family Health Strategies (ESF) teams in the 2nd Sanitary District of Maceio-AL, who work as preceptors, i.e. professionals from the service who receive students from the HEI, with the ESF as a practice setting for the students' training.

4.3 Location

UNCISAL classrooms and community spaces in the communities where the professionals are based.

4.4 Objectives

3.4.1 General Objective

To train the preceptors of the II Sanitary District of Maceio in the theory and interdisciplinary practice of the Family Health Strategy.

4.4.2 Specific Objectives

Get to know the daily practices of the preceptors with regard to Interdisciplinarity;

To understand how students participate in the collective activities of the ESF;

Carry out theoretical and practical experiences on interdisciplinarity;

Propose a reorganization of collective support in the ESF with a more integrative approach.

4.5 Goals

Better understanding of the concept and practice of interdisciplinarity on the part of the preceptors, realizing that through interdisciplinarity, comprehensive health care is achieved, in accordance with the SUS guidelines.

Drawing up, applying and evaluating interdisciplinary proposals during training.

4.6 Performance Period

July and August 2013, with the proposal of a weekly meeting, which could be agreed with the participants.

4.7 Methodology

Initially, the HEI, through PROEG (Pro-Rectory for Teaching and Graduation), will locate the preceptors for the II Health District of Maceio. This can be done at the Family Health Strategy Sector located at the Municipal Health Department. The preceptors should then be invited to the training. Seven moments are suggested:

1) The first meeting will be one of socializing and listening, in which each professional will introduce themselves, talk about their practices in the ESFs and the participation of the students. On this day, there will be an initial introduction to the topic. Each participant will write or draw something that represents interdisciplinarity. Groups will then be formed with different professional categories to discuss and draw a new picture with the aim of uniting ideas and building a new idea, a new picture that represents interdisciplinarity. Finally, on this day, the concept will be introduced through texts on "Interdisciplinarity". The texts will be discussed at the same time as the drawings.
2) Theoretical deepening on the subject in a participatory and dialogical way. The professional responsible for conducting this session must be from the HEI and will initially provide a listening session so that the preceptors can tell us what they know about the subject of interdisciplinarity. This will be followed by a presentation of the topic "Interdisciplinary Theory and Practice", based on reference literature on

the subject, allowing for participation and dialogue with the preceptors during the presentation.

3) Study of scientific articles on the subject, discussion and deepening of the concept of *interdisciplinarity.*
4) Division of support groups, made up of different professional categories, which may be in the same ESF. At this meeting, each group will discuss and propose a collective and shared action, with a common goal, from an interdisciplinary perspective, taking into account the assisted community and the needs existing in each one, including the participation of students.
5) Implementation of the interdisciplinary proposal in Family Health Strategies.
6) Final Seminar. Presentation (video, slides, photographs) and sharing of support in the large group. At this point, in addition to presenting the interdisciplinary proposal, the motivations, difficulties and strategies used to carry out the interdisciplinary practice will be presented.
7) Finalization with the return of the initial proposal for the construction of the concept through the drawing/symbol of interdisciplinarity for each team. Follow-up and agreement for possible new training.

4.8 Products and/or Expected Results

It is hoped that the project's objectives will be achieved, especially with regard to the understanding of the professional preceptors of the II Sanitary District of Maceio regarding interdisciplinary theory and practice in the Family Health Strategy. It is believed that the preceptors will be the main multipliers of interdisciplinary support in their Family Health teams.

4.9 Schedule

Date/Time	Proposed Activities
05.07.2013/14h	Socializing and listening to the theme.
12.07.2013/14h	Deepening the theory of "Interdisciplinarity".
19.07.2013/14h	Case studies.
26.07.2013/14h	Division of the action/reflection groups and preparation of the interdisciplinary proposal.
Day of the week and time chosen by the team	Implementation of the interdisciplinary proposal in the practice settings.
16.08.2013/14h	Final Seminar
23.08.2013/14h	Finalization, monitoring and agreement.

4.10 Organization

Consumables	Amount in R$
Standard printer ink	59,90
Ream of A4 paper	14,90
Copies	19,00
Stapler	19,90
Ballpoint pen	6,00
Graphite pencil (ordinary)	3,00
Rubber	1,50
Binding	15,00
Total value	79,30

4.11 Monitoring and Evaluation

The evaluation will be continuous and progressive, on a weekly basis, emphasizing that learning should reflect all this knowledge and will be based on meeting the objectives, culminating in the last meeting. With this training, it is hoped that the preceptors will have achieved the proposed training objectives and strengthened their bond with the HEI.

It is hoped that monitoring by the HEI will continue after the training has taken place, and that this monitoring will take place on a permanent basis, both in theory, through academic meetings, and in practice, in the services in which the students work. We also believe that the training is a support and an awakening to the practice of interdisciplinarity.

REFERENCES

BARRETO, V. H. et al. Role of the primary health care preceptor in undergraduate and postgraduate training at the Federal University of Pernambuco - a Term of Reference. **Rev. Bras. Educ. Med.**, v. 35, n. 4, p. 578-583, 2011.

BRAZIL. Law no. 8.080, of September 19, 1990. Provides on the conditions for the promotion, protection and recovery of health, the organization and operation of the corresponding services and other measures. **Diario Oficial [da] Republica Federativa do Brasil**, Poder Legislativo, Brasilia, DF, September 20, 1990, Section 1, p. 18055.

. Ordinance No. 648/GM, of March 28, 2006. National Primary Care Policy. Disposes of the guidelines and norms for the organization of Basic Care. **Diario Oficial [da] Republica Federativa do** Brasil, Brasilia, DF, March 28, 2006. Section 1, p 71.

BOTTI, S.; REGO, S. Preceptor, supervisor, tutor and mentor: what are their roles? **Rev. Bras. Educ. Med**. v. 32. n. 3, p. 363-373, 2008.

CECCIM, R.B.; FEUERWEKER, L. C. M. The quadrilateral of health training: teaching, management, care and social control. **Physis: Rev. Saude Coletiva**, Rio de Janeiro, v.14, n.1, jan./jun., p. 41-65, 2004a.

ROSA, W. A. G; LABATE, R. C. Family Health Program: building a new model of care. **Rev. Latino Americana de Enfermagem**. Sao Paulo, v. 13, n. 6, p.1027-34, 2005.

5 GENERAL CONCLUSION

This work presented field research and a product in the form of an intervention project in line with the study. Both the research and the product had *interdisciplinarity* as their central object.

The survey data showed that the preceptors were unfamiliar with interdisciplinarity, both in terms of theory and interdisciplinary practice. As a suggestion for improving work in the ESF, the preceptors suggested training on the subject of interdisciplinarity, entitled: "Interdisciplinarity in Health Teaching: Reframing collective support through a shared and integrated approach".

The conclusions drawn from this work do not exhaust the subject in question. It is believed that there are many factors that make it impossible to practice interdisciplinarity, such as personal motivation, academic training, interpersonal relationships and the individual search for professional qualification. Health professionals need to understand that in order to put integrality into practice, a guideline advocated by the SUS, it is through the interaction and cooperation of disciplines in the search for new knowledge. This new knowledge will enable the integral vision that the new curriculum guidelines indicate for the training of health professionals.

Furthermore, interdisciplinarity can help to overcome the dissociation of the knowledge produced and guide the production of a new order of knowledge, which is a necessary condition for improving health training for the SUS. It is believed that other influences and aspects can and should be considered with regard to interdisciplinarity. Therefore, this research points to new and productive studies.

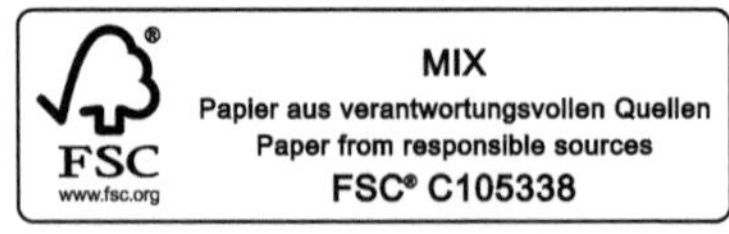

Printed by Books on Demand GmbH, Norderstedt / Germany